# Understanding
# THE MENO

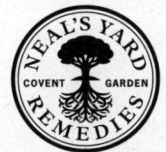

Imprint

Neal's Yard Press, 16 Stambourne Way, West Wickham, Kent BR4 9NF,
e-mail: menopause@winterpress.net

Conceived and produced by Winter Press, for Neal's Yard Press,
Text and artwork © 2008


ISBN 978-1-905830-305
Printed by PrintRite, West Wickham, BR4.

All rights reserved. No part of this publication may be reproduced, stored in a retrieval system, or transmitted, in any form or by any means, electronic, mechanical, photocopying, recording or otherwise, without the prior permission of Winter Press.

This book is presented as a collection of natural remedies and as an aid in understanding their use. It is not intended to replace or supersede professional consultation or treatment and no guarantee can be given as to the efficacy or appropriateness of a remedy in an individual case without professional advice.

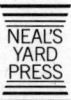

# CONTENTS

| | |
|---|---|
| 2 | INTRODUCTION |
| 3 | ALTERNATIVES TO HRT |
| 4 | A HEALTHY MENOPAUSE |
| 6 | THE MENOPAUSE TRANSITION |
| 8 | HRT |
| 10 | HOT FLUSHES |
| 14 | VAGINAL/GENITAL PROBLEMS |
| 17 | ANXIETY AND DEPRESSION |
| 21 | OSTEOPOROSIS |
| 24 | HORMONAL BALANCING FORMULA |
| 25 | HRT CAKE |
| 26 | DETOX DIET |
| 28 | SYMPTOMS CHECKLIST |
| 29 | REFERENCES |

# Introduction

In the decade before 2003 the number of women opting for Hormone Replacement Therapy (HRT) to relieve symptoms of the menopause was increasing rapidly; but then the results of a study into the link between an increased risk of developing breast cancer and taking HRT were published in the Journal of the American Medical Association (JAMA)[1]. As the Guardian newspaper headline of 8th August 2003 read, "HRT treatment doubles the risk of breast cancer".

Since then the number of prescriptions of HRT have understandably plummeted. Studies two or more years on from the decline is use have shown a decrease in the number of new breast cancer cases. This strongly supports the link between the hormonal therapy and an increased risk of developing cancer.[2,3]

---

1    Journal of the American Medical Association, June 25th 2003
2    University of Texas research (BBC News Online, December 15th 2006)
3    Katalinic A, Rawal R. Decline in breast cancer incidence after decrease in utilisation of hormone replacement therapy, Breast Cancer Research & Treatment, 2008 Feb;107(3):427-30

# Alternatives to HRT

There are many natural remedies that are effective treatments for all the symptoms that may accompany the menopause, including hot flushes, heavy menstruation, vaginitis, anxiety, depression and osteoporosis. This booklet will help you to choose the most appropriate remedies for your particular symptoms. It also gives you an easy to follow detox program that will help to eliminate toxins from the system and improve the function of the liver. If you follow the guidelines the remedies are safe to use and will enhance your health rather than undermine it.

Some of us have deeper health problems than others, and it is advisable to seek professional help from a qualified practitioner:

- if you have been on HRT for a number of years and want to come off it or mitigate any damage it may have caused
- if any of your symptoms do not respond within a few months of treating yourself
- if menopausal symptoms are part of a bigger picture of poor health
- if you have concerns after reading the symptoms checklist on page 28

The Contacts on page 29 will help you to find a suitable practitioner.

# A Healthy Menopause

The menopause is potentially one of the most liberating transitions in every woman's life.

It can herald a shift to greater freedom and personal satisfaction as you move from constantly supplying family needs to having more time and space to express your own purpose. Making love can also become more relaxed and adventurous as the fear of pregnancy recedes.

## Other Cultures

In more traditional societies the role of the older woman is well established in the community, and such things as wisdom, calmness and more time to observe and reflect are valued and respected. From an energetic perspective during the fertile years a woman's spiritual energy ebbs and flows during her menstrual cycle, after the menopause the spiritual contact can be more direct and consistent.

There are still societies where the cessation of periods that indicates the menopause physically, is just that and no other symptoms are expected. Japanese women, for example, are known for their lack of menopausal symptoms such as hot flushes, attributed mainly to their increased consumption of soya based products, which are high in phytoestrogens.[4]

---

[4] Toohey, L.; ed, Nutri Notes, 1998;Vol 3;No 6.

# A New Phase of Life

In western society ageing has become associated with failure and losing one's function, becoming less useful and unattractive. The emphasis on youthful appearance has led to a great fear among many women of showing the natural signs of ageing and embracing one's changing role and status.

The key to a healthy menopause is to accept it as a time of transition into a new phase of life and not view it as the beginning of a decline. There are many positive examples of women at this stage of their lives who have changed careers, moved to a different part of the country or chosen to pursue their own interest in such things as a natural medicine course, gardening or painting.

## Positive Help

If you are finding it difficult to have a positive attitude towards this major life transition then the Australian Bush Flower Essence called Woman Essence can be very helpful.

It has been developed to encourage a woman's own innate strength and beauty and it will help to harmonize mood swings and balance the emotions during the menopause. Simply take a few drops morning and night for a few weeks.

# The Menopause Transition

Like all periods of transition, the menopause can throw up symptoms both emotionally and physically as we move through it.

The average age of the menopause is 52 (although anything between 48 and 54 is normal and many woman may be younger), and the cessation of periods is the observable result of a number of complex hormonal changes occurring within the body.

The ovaries, the pituitary and the hypothalamus in the brain are the glands that communicate with each other to regulate the menstrual cycle. During menopause the hormonal balance begins to change, and less oestrogen produced by the ovaries.

At around the same time, more follicle stimulating hormone (FSH) and luteinizing hormone (LH) are produced by the pituitary. It is usually the level of FSH that is measured when testing for the menopause occurring. These hormonal changes, when out of balance, are responsible for the symptoms such as hot flushes and night sweats that can occur during the menopause.

The decline in oestrogen fluctuates at first, but eventually tapers off. This is then replaced by a form of oestrogen called oestrone, that is converted from androgen mainly produced by the adrenal glands. Insufficient oestrogen can lead to the symptoms of hot flushes, vaginal dryness and in the longer term, osteoporosis. This emphasises the importance of having healthy adrenal glands if we want to enjoy good health after the menopause. The adrenal glands are especially prone to damage by poor nutrition and an excess of stress.

## What goes wrong?

The liver has the job of breaking down 'old' hormones and eliminating them from the body. If the liver is not functioning efficiently then these 'old' hormones continue to circulate in the body causing PMT-like symptoms, hot flushes, irritability and headaches and can eventually lead to a range of tumours such as fibroids and, when malignant, to cancer. Going on a detox program can really help the liver to regenerate and this is why a regular detox can be the key to reducing menopausal symptoms (see page 26).

## External factors

Xenoestrogens are literally 'foreign oestrogens' that come from certain chemicals commonly found in pesticides and some plastics.

It is the prevalence of xenoestrogens in recent years that is thought to be responsible for the earlier onset of puberty and they are increasingly being linked to certain cancers, especially breast cancer[5]. This again stresses the importance of having a healthy functioning liver as it is the liver that will detoxify the body of the xenoestrogens. It also underlines the importance of having a healthy diet based on organically produced foods to reduce exposure to pesticide residues.

## Artificially induced menopause

Medically induced menopause and hysterectomy are more frequently used these days to treat conditions such as endometriosis and uterine fibroids. The symptoms experienced are the same as those in natural menopause. While the symptoms are reversible in drug induced menopause once the medication is discontinued, bone thinning may have occurred during treatment. It would be beneficial to make some of the nutritional and lifestyle modifications discussed later to prevent this.

Inducing menopause artificially can be inadvertent, perhaps during radiotherapy – particularly to the pelvic region. The herb Dong Quai (*Angelica sinensis*) may be used to help protect the ovary during treatment.[6]

---

5   Massart F, et al. "How do environmental estrogen disruptors induce precocious puberty?" Minerva Pediatr. 2006 Jun;58(3):247-54
6   Trickey R, Women, Hormones & The Menstrual Cycle, Allen & Unwin 2003

# HRT

Hormone Replacement Therapy introduces synthetic hormones into the bloodstream to replace the oestrogen supplies that are waning naturally as part of the menopausal process.

Initially HRT was based on oestrogen only but research results quickly showed that this led to an increased risk of cancer of the uterus.[7] Oestrogen alone causes a build up of the lining of the womb, and mutations were occurring in these endometrial cells.

Then progesterone was added to cause a regular bleed and the combined oestrogen progesterone HRT became the most popular treatment. Combined HRT has become routinely prescribed for women concerned about any symptoms of the menopause or even just to keep more youthful looking. What started out as a medical treatment rapidly became a lifestyle choice used by millions of women in the developed world.

However, in June 2003 the Journal of the American Medical Association (JAMA) published a study showing that the risk of breast cancer doubles in women who take combined HRT. The authors stated that, "In the meantime, the message for physicians caring for menopausal patients is clear. The increased risk of breast cancer and the mammographic abnormalities among women in the WHI study provide further compelling evidence against the use of combination estrogen plus progestin hormone therapy."

---

[7] Hoover, R., et al, New England Journal of Medicine, 1976:Vol 295:401-5

## How do I come off HRT?

If you have been on HRT for more than two years, it is advisable to come off HRT with the help of a qualified practitioner. They will be able to work with you to alleviate any symptoms that may arise when you stop taking it, including the original symptoms that may have been the reason for you starting it. A natural practitioner will also be able to put you on a program to help reduce the potentially damaging effects of having been on HRT for a lengthy period of time.

If you have been on HRT for less than two years you can come off it and use the natural remedies, such as those described in this book to help you deal with any uncomfortable symptoms of the menopause. If your original symptoms were severe, or if you try the remedies and they do not seem to help then you will need to consult a qualified practitioner to help you find alternatives that suit you. In addition to the suggestions discussed here – from aromatherapy, herbalism and nutrition – the therapies of homœopathy and acupuncture and others may also be of great benefit.

# Hot Flushes

Hot flushes are one of the most common symptoms women experience during the menopause, they occur in an estimated 80% of women in the west.[8] A rush of heat passes over the chest, neck and face causing redness and perspiration. They may also occur at night, although often the woman wakes drenched in sweat when the hot flush itself has passed, and are called 'night sweats'. Many women only experience one or two a month, but some women can have as many as 15 or 20 hot flushes a day which becomes very debilitating.

---

8   Ammer, C., The A-Z of Women's Health, 1983, Harper Collins: London.

Hot flushes most commonly begin to appear when oestrogen levels begin to taper off at the onset of menopause and can continue for several years after the last period, although they will stop of their own accord once the body readjusts to not having oestrogen in the system. It is believed they are caused by a disturbance to the hypothalamus gland as it attempts to readjust to the change in hormone levels. Severe hot flushes can result from the surgical removal of the ovaries.

Hot flushes are greatly relieved by HRT and are one of the chief reasons for taking HRT, although they will usually return in force when HRT is stopped and the body has to go through the period of readjustment again.

Lifestyle measures that can help to relieve the impact of hot flushes include wearing several layers of clothing, so that layers can be removed when over-heated. Alcohol and spicy food can both bring on hot flushes and so may be best avoided at this stage of a woman's life.

There are a number of natural remedies for hot flushes, some of which have now undergone impressive clinical trials showing their effectiveness. See which of the following seem best indicated.

## Herbs

These may be taken as infusions, liquid extracts (tinctures) or capsules.

SAGE (SALVIA OFFICINALIS) – This is one of the most important herbs for relieving hot flushes. In a recent clinical trial the herbal tincture showed a reduction in hot flushes by 56% when taken over an 8 week period.[9]

---

9   De Leo, V., Lanzette, D., Cazzavacca, R., Morgante, G., "Treatment of Neurovegetative Menopausal Symptoms with a Phytotherapeutic Agent", 1998: Minerva Ginecol;50 (5):207-11.

CHASTEBERRY (VITEX AGNUS CASTUS) – Is a hormonal regulator that can help to relieve hot flushes by balancing the hormones.[10] It may be combined with sage.

## Essential Oils

These may be diluted in a massage oil base to massage into the skin, or a bath oil to add to the bath.

CYPRESS – Is a cooling and refreshing essential oil that can help to relieve excessive sweating and hot flushes.

GERANIUM – Is cooling and will help to relieve hot flushes by having a balancing action on the hormones.

CLARY SAGE – Can help to reduce excessive perspiration and hot flushes.

## Nutrition

BIOFLAVONOIDS – Supplements containing bioflavonoid complex combined with Vitamin C have successfully reduced hot flushes in trials.[11]

VITAMIN E – A number of studies have shown supplements of this vitamin to be helpful in reducing hot flushes.[12]

---

10   Milewicz, A., Gejdel, E., Sworen, H., Sienkiewicz, K., Jedrzejak, J., Teucher, T., Schmitz, H., "Vitex Agnus Castus extract in the treatment of luteal phase defects due to latent hyperprolactinemia", 1993: Arneimittelforschung 43 (7):752-6.
11   Smith, C.J., "Non-hormonal control of vaso-motor flushing in menopausal patients", 1964: Chicago Medicine.
12   McLaren, H., "Vitamin E in the Menopause", 1949: British Medical Journal; 1378-82.

PHYTOESTROGENS – Phytoestrogens are plant derived compounds that have similar structure to oestrogens, which gives them the ability to bind to oestrogen receptors, but their ostrogen activity is relatively low.[13] Once they bind to the receptor they can have either an oestrogenic or anti-ostrogenic affect depending on whether the individual is pre or post menopause.

The most potent form of phytoestrogens are called isoflavones and include soya[14] and red clover which been found to alleviate menopausal symptoms including hot flushes.[15,16]

Soya may be incorporated into your diet in teh form of soya milk, soya flour or derived soya products such as tofu. Soya food supplements, taken to relieve menopausal symtoms, area lso available. To relieve hot flushes red clover is best taken in capsule form as a food supplement.

Other dietary sources of phytostrogens are linseeds, black/green tea, many fruits and vegetables, split peas, lentils and beans. And another common category called coumestans is found in alfalfa, beans, split peas and lentils.

---

13. Pengelly, A, 2004, The Constituents of Medicinal Plants, 2nd Edition, Allen & Unwin NSW
14   Journal of Nutrition, 1995:Vol 125;437-45
15   Hidalgo LA et al. The effect of red clover isoflavones on menopausal symptoms, lipids and vaginal cytology in menopausal women: a randomized, double-blind, placebo-controlled study. Gynecol Endocrinol, 2005 Nov; 21(5):257-64.
16   Messina M & Hughes C. Efficacy of Soyfoods and Soybean Isoflavone Supplements for Alleviating Menopausal Symptoms Is Positively Related to Initial Hot Flush Frequency, Journal of Medicinal Food. March 1, 2003, 6(1): 1-11

# Vaginal/Genital Problems

The decline in oestrogen that occurs during the menopause leads to a thinning, drying and loss of elasticity in the tissues of the vulva and vagina.

A few years after the periods have stopped, the vagina walls will have become thinner and less mucus is produced. This can result in painful sexual intercourse and also in a greater tendency to genital itching (pruritis) and vaginal and urinary infections (cystitis).

Not all women experience problems of this nature, and the response seems to be highly individual. Lots of women continue to enjoy an active sex life for many years after the menopause, and there are a number of measures that can be taken to improve the quality of the vaginal tissue. General steps include wearing natural fibres such as cotton underwear and loose clothing to reduce the likelihood of vaginal itching and infections. Using a lubricant such as KY Jelly or aloe vera juice before intercourse can be helpful.

The following remedies have all been shown to be helpful for vaginal problems. (See also the Hormonal Balancing Formula on page 24)

## Herbs

These may be taken as infusions, liquid extracts (tinctures) or capsules.

BLACK COHOSH (CIMICIFUGA RACEMOSA) – This herb has a high phytoestrogen content and is particularly useful in helping to relieve symptoms of vaginal dryness.[17]

---

17   Stolze, H., "An alternative to treat menopausal symptoms", Gynaecology, 1982:Vol 3;14-16.

DONG QUAI (ANGELICA SINENSIS) – This is a traditional Chinese herbal tonic for the female reproductive system. It can be helpful in relieving symptoms of vaginal dryness.[18]

## Essential Oils

These should be diluted in a base oil to use in the bath or added to an ointment base to apply to the genital area.

CHAMOMILE – A soothing and anti-inflammatory essential oil particularly useful for relieving vaginal itching or irritation.[19]

GERANIUM – Has a cooling action and helps to balance the hormones. Regular use may be helpful for vaginal irritation.[20]

LAVENDER – A soothing, antiseptic and anti-inflammatory essential oil that can be used to relieve the symptoms of vaginal irritation or infections.[21]

ROSE – A profoundly soothing and nourishing oil that also has aphrodisiac properties. May be used to help relieve the symptoms of vaginal dryness and painful intercourse.

SANDALWOOD – A particularly useful oil for soothing dry, inflamed mucous membranes of the genital area. May be blended with Rose or other appropriate essential oils.

---

18  Balch, J.F & Balch, P.A, "Prescription for Nutritional Healing", 1990: Avery Publishing;NY.
19  Grgsania, D., Mandic, M.L., Kanisa, L., Klapec, T., Bockinac, D., "Chemical composition of different parts of Matricaria chamomilla", 1995: Prehambeno Tehnoloska I Biotehnoloska Revija 33, 2-3, 111-113.
20  Bard, M., Albrecht, M.R., Gupta, N., Guynn, C.J., Stillwell, W., "Geraniol interferes with membrane functions in strains of Candida and Saccharomyces", 1998: Lipids,23,6,534-538.
21  Hili, P., "Antimicrobial Properties of Essential Oils", 2001: Winter Press, Kent..

# Nutrition

Essential fatty acids (EFAs) will help to keep the body's tissues, including those of the vagina more elastic and well-lubricated and need to be incorporated into the diet. They are found in oily fish and many nuts, seeds and vegetable oils which should be eaten on a regular basis in addition to considering the supplements below.

### FLAX SEED OIL
Rich in EFAs that will help to keep the vagina more elastic and well-lubricated. May be used as an oil in dressings or taken in capsule form.

### VITAMIN E
An important vitamin for the health of the genitals, one study has shown that 50% of women taking 400iu Vitamin E capsules internally for vaginal dryness were helped.[22] The oil may also be used externally to lubricate the vagina.

### PHYTOESTROGENS
These plant-based hormones can help to buffer the effects of declining oestrogen. Add more soya products, cabbage and fennel to the diet and consider taking a phytoestrogen supplement.[23]

### PROBIOTICS
These 'friendly' bacteria increase the effectiveness of phytoestrogen function[24] and also will help to prevent thrush and other vaginal infections developing.

---

22  Glenville, M., "The Natural Health Handbook for Women", 2001, Piatkus, London
23  Hidalgo LA et al. The effect of red clover isoflavones on menopausal symptoms, lipids and vaginal cytology in menopausal women: a randomized, double-blind, placebo-controlled study. Gynecol Endocrinol, 2005 Nov; 21(5):257-64.
24  Advances in Experimental Medicine and Biology AICR, 1996:401;63-99.

# Anxiety and Depression

Some women experience an increase in symptoms such as irritability, anxiety, fatigue and depression during the menopause.

Such symptoms are certainly not inevitable and many women feel that the psychological and physical aspects of the menopause are overstated.[25] However, in other women the symptoms of anxiety and depression are more severe and can be a reason for considering HRT.

If you do suffer with menopausal anxiety and depression it will probably respond best to a dual psychological and physical therapy approach. A re-evaluation of priorities and purpose may be necessary and changes in lifestyle required before you can achieve a sense of well-being again. Professional guidance such as one of the many types of counselling, or flower remedy therapy may be helpful although for some women a period of focussed individual reflection may be sufficient. More severe psychological symptoms should always be referred to a professional practitioner for assessment.

### THE ADRENAL POWERHOUSE

The key area of physical health to work on if suffering with symptoms such as fatigue, poor concentration and depression during the menopause is the adrenals. The adrenal glands supply us with the hormones that provide our energy and enthusiasm for life. As the ovaries begin to supply less oestrogen during the menopause, we rely on the adrenals even more for oestrone – an oestrogen-like hormone. If the adrenals are depleted then we will suffer with a lack of energy, libido and lack of optimism.

The adrenals also supply the hormone cortisol which helps provide endurance and feelings of stability, if the adrenals are not supplying cortisol efficiently then mood swings and anxiety will result.

---

25  Journal of Health and Social Behaviour, 1987:28(4);345-63.

The adrenals are sensitive to damage from both emotional stress and physical or environmental stress. Caffeine is particularly damaging to the adrenals and should be avoided if you suffer any of these symptoms.[26]

SUPPORTIVE STEPS
The following suggestions are known to help support the adrenals or provide support for symptoms such as anxiety during the menopause.

If you have a very stressful lifestyle then improvement may only be obtained by making changes to it. Also if your general level of health is very poor, and it is likely that your adrenals are severely depleted then seeing a qualified practitioner will be necessary.

There are laboratories which can measure your hormone levels, including those secreted by the adrenals, and in more severe cases it may be advisable to visit a practitioner who can arrange for these tests and appropriate treatment. See the list of Contacts at the back of the booklet for more information.

# Herbs

These may be taken as infusions, liquid extracts (tinctures) or capsules.

ST JOHN'S WORT – This is a herb that is traditionally used to treat menopausal anxiety and depression. Clinical trials have recently demonstrated that it helps relieve psychological symptoms of the menopause including irritability, poor concentration, tension, anxiety and depression.[27] It was also shown to help enhance sexual well-being for menopausal women.

You could try taking a combination of St John's wort with black cohosh as clinical trials have found the combination of black cohosh

---

26  Northrup, C., "Women's Bodies Women's Wisdom", 1998, Piatkus: London.
27  Grube, B., Walper, A., Wheatley, D., "St John's wort extract: efficacy for menopausal symptoms of psychological origin", Advances in Therapy, 1999: 16(4):177-186.

and St. John's wort to be superior to black cohosh alone in alleviating mood symptoms in menopause.[28]

VERVAIN – A herb that acts as a tonic to the nervous system and the endocrine glands. Helps to relieve symptoms of anxiety, tension and stress including headaches, insomnia, irritability and depression. Vervain may be taken in combination with St John's wort and black cohosh

## Essential Oils

These may be diluted in a massage oil base to massage into the skin on a daily basis, or a bath oil to add to the bath.

GERANIUM – An uplifting essential oil that has a balancing action on the hormones and emotions. Useful for symptoms of tension and irritability.

LAVENDER – A profoundly soothing and relaxing essential oil. Useful for symptoms of anxiety, insomnia and tension. Will help to relieve headaches and panic attacks.

NEROLI – An uplifting essential oil with an anti-depressant action. Useful for treating anxiety, depression, stress and fatigue.

ROSE – A profoundly feminine oil that helps to nurture feelings of self-worth. Has an anti-depressant and balancing action on the emotions.

---

28 Briese V et al., "Black cohosh with or without St. John's wort for symptom-specific climacteric treatment--results of a large-scale, controlled, observational study". Maturitas. 2007 Aug 20;57(4):405-14

# Nutrition

OATS – An excellent tonic for the nervous system, oats can help relieve depression, nervousness, anxiety and stress. Eat as muesli or porridge daily. May also be taken as an herbal tincture in combination with other tinctures.[29]

B VITAMINS – Essential for a healthy nervous system, B vitamins help to reduce the impact of stress on the body. They are found naturally in wholegrain cereals, pulses and yeast extract. A supplement of B vitamin complex can be beneficial to relieve symptoms of stress, anxiety and tension.

TRYPTOPHAN – Called by some an alternative to HRT because of its ability to improve bone density, depression and relieve hot flushes.[30]

Tryptophan and 5-Hydroxytryptophan (5-HTP) are naturally occurring amino acids (found in protein) necessary for the formation of Serotonin, a feel good chemical in the body, deficiency of which can lead to depression and anxiety, common symptoms in menopause.

Tryptophan and 5-HTP have been shown in clinical trials to enhance the synthesis of serotonin and thus alleviate depression and anxiety. It is suggested that increasing serotonin in the diet may also alleviate the hot flushes associated with menopause.[31]

Food sources of tryptophan are cheese, chicken, eggs, fish, milk, nuts, peanut butter, peanuts, pumpkin seeds, sesame seeds., soy, tofu and turkey.[32] For a therapeutic dose a supplement may be necessary. There are plenty of 5-HTP supplements available on the market.

---

29   Curtis, S., Fraser, R., "Natural Healing for Women", 2003, Thorsons: London.
30   Richards JB et al., "Effect of selective serotonin reuptake inhibitors on the risk of fracture". Arch Intern Med. 2007 Jan 22;167(2):188-94
31   Curcio JJ, Kim LS, Wollner D, Pockaj BA, The potential of 5-hydryoxytryptophan for hot flash reduction: a hypothesis. Altern Med Rev. 2005 Sep;10(3):216-21
32   University of Maryland Medical Centre

# Osteoporosis

Osteoporosis is a skeletal disease where the bone mass declines and the bone structure deteriorates. As a consequence, there is an increase in bone fragility and in susceptibility to fracture.

A decline in oestrogen is one of the potential factors leading to osteoporosis, and this is one of the main reasons for prescribing HRT. However, HRT only protects against osteoporosis for as long as it is taken, and users of HRT will steadily 'catch up' with non-users once they stop taking it. Given the increased risk of other diseases, such as breast cancer, from taking HRT it makes more sense to adopt the other lifestyle and nutritional changes that can prevent or slow down the progress of osteoporosis.

## Exercise

Physical exercise is a key factor in the prevention of osteoporosis, and moderate exercise has even been shown to increase the bone mass in postmenopausal women.[33] It is the duration of the exercise that is as important as the intensity, and walking is a good exercise to start with. A 45 minute walk at least three times a week is an example of the level of exercise that is required.[34] Weight bearing exercises, the kind of activities that move against gravity while standing upright, are the best for building bone strength.[35] Examples of weight- bearing exercises include walking, jogging, dancing, stair climbing, hiking, low impact aerobics, tennis, etc.

---

33  Yeater, R., Martin, R., "Senile osteoporosis: the effects of exercise", Postgraduate Medicine, 1984:75;174-9.
34  Murray, M., Pizzorno, J., "Encyclopaedia of Natural Medicine", 1990, Little, Brown: London.
35  National Osteoporosis Foundation

# Nutrition

Good nutrition is a key factor to maintaining healthy bones throughout life; a varied diet with plenty of whole grains, seeds, nuts, fresh fruit and vegetables is essential.

Poor diets with low intakes of dairy products and fruits and vegetables compromise the intakes of other nutrients essential for bone health.36 Nutrients including calcium, potassium, magnesium and vitamin D are all necessary for optimal bone health. Other nutrients also necessary are vitamins A, C, E and K and minerals phosphorus, fluoride, iron, zinc, copper and boron. In addition the diet should consist of adequate intake of alkaline rich foods (fresh fruit and vegetables) with moderate protein and limited salt, caffeine, fizzy drinks, sugar and alcohol.[37]

It is well documented that oestrogen can prevent bone loss.[38] However up until now this had been treated with HRT which has since been linked to the development of breast cancer. Phytoestrogens can also positively effect oestrogen levels in the body. However, unlike HRT, phytoestrogens, in particular isolflavones such as soy and black cohosh are believed to act on receptors in the body predominately found in bone and vascular tissue, rather than tissue in the breast or ovaries.[39] This would suggest that they are a safer alternative. Recent interest in phytoestrogens has lead to clinical trials indicating that black cohosh extracts are also effective in protecting against postmenopausal bone loss.[40]

---

36  Richardson, D., "Nutrition in Transition", CRN:UK, September 2002.
37  Miggiano GA & Gagliardi L. 'Diet, nutrition and bone health' Clin Ter. 2005 Jan-Apr;156(1-2):47-56
38  Fogelman I., Oestrogen, the prevention of bone loss and osteoporosis. Br J Rheumatol. 1991 Aug;30(4):276-81
39  Mason P, 'How effective are complementary therapies for menopausal symptoms?', The Pharmaceutical Journal 2004 Vol. 273
40  Chan et al, Ethanolic extract of Actaea racemosa (black cohosh) potentiates bone nodule formation in MC3T3-E1 preosteoblast cells. Bone. 2008 Sep;43(3):567-73

Food sources of calcium are salmon and sardines, shellfish, almonds, brazil nuts, and dried beans. Rich sources of magnesium include tofu, legumes, whole grains, green leafy vegetables, wheat bran, brazil nuts, soybean flour, almonds, cashews, blackstrap molasses, pumpkin and squash seeds, pine nuts, and walnuts.[41]

## VITAMIN D

This vitamin is essential for the efficient utilisation of calcium in the body. Vitamin D deficiency has been implicated in bone fractures in women regardless of age.[42] It is considered that the best source of vitamin D is from sun exposure, which should be taken in 15 minute intervals, 3 times a week in the summer and a supplement in the winter time.[43]

Concerns about the ageing and skin-damaging effects of over exposure to the sun have caused many to always use sun screens and cover up in the sun. As a result an increasing number of women with vitamin D deficieny are being seen. We need to develop a balanced approach for a healthy level of exposure to sunlight without casusing skin damage.

---

41  University of Maryland Medical Centre
42  Steele B. et al., "Vitamin D Deficiency: A Common Occurrence in Both High- and Low-energy Fractures", HSS J. 2008 Sep;4(2):143-8
43  www.anhcampaign.org, 'Vitamin D: as close to a magic bullet as you can get?' Sep 2008

# Supplements

## CALCIUM & MAGNESIUM

These are best taken in combination as both are needed to prevent bone loss. Studies show that oral supplementation with calcium and magnesium combined can help to prevent bone loss and increase the re-mineralisation of bone tissue in post-menopausal women.[44]

## BORON

A mineral which has been found to play a role in bone formation[45] and is now widely used in bone formula supplements. Its has also been found to elevate oestradiol levels (a form of oestrogen).[46] Dried prunes are an great source of boron, with just a serving of prunes (100 g) fulfilling the daily requirement (2 to 3 mg).[47]

---

44  Abraham, G., Grewal, H., "A total dietary program emphasizing magnesium instead of calcium", Journal of Reproductive Medicine, 1990:35;503-507.
45  Miggiano GA, Gagliardi L. Diet, nutrition and bone health, Clin Ter. 2005 Jan-Apr;156(1-2):47-56
46  FH Nielsen, CD Hunt, LM Mullen and JR Hunt , 'Effect of dietary boron on mineral, estrogen, and testosterone metabolism in postmenopausal women', The FASEB Journal, Vol 1, 394-397
47  Stacewicz-Sapuntzakis M et al, Chemical composition and potential health effects of prunes: a functional food? Crit Rev Food Sci Nutr. 2001 May;41(4):251-86

# Hormonal Balancing Formula

The following formula is a combination of herbal tinctures developed by the herbalist Dragana Vilinac to take during the menopause. It combines herbs that are tonic to the endocrine glands, reproductive organs and nervous system. It will help to reduce hot flushes, relieve fatigue and depression, increase libido and have a phytoestrogen action.

This formula is an excellent general tonic to balance the hormones and should be taken for a minimum of 3 months. It is not suitable to take if you are on anticoagulant drugs eg. Warfarin, or during pregnancy. If you take any other medication consult a qualified practitioner before taking it. See the list of Contacts at the back of the booklet to locate suppliers of this formula. At Neal's Yard Remedies it is available ready blended as Black Cohosh and Sage Formula. Take 2-4ml three times daily. Start by taking the lower dose and gradually build up to the higher dose over the period of 2-3 weeks.

| PLANT SPECIES | QUANTITY |
| --- | --- |
| *Black Cohosh (Cimicifuga racemosa)* | 20 ml |
| *Chasteberry (Vitex agnus castus)* | 15 ml |
| *Dong Quai – Chinese Angelica (Angelica sinensis)* | 15 ml |
| *Schizandra Fruit – Wu Wei Zi (Schisandra chinensis)* | 20 ml |
| *Sage (Salvia officinalis)* | 10 ml |
| *Vervain (Verbena officinalis)* | 20 ml |

Rehmania Root (*Rehmania glutinosa*, prepared root) – Add this if your hot flushes are excessive, either take 1ml 3 times a day or add 10 ml to mixture above.

# HRT Cake

This recipe contains lots of ingredients rich in phytoestrogens. It is a very tasty way of eating the foods like soya and linseed that are renowned to help reduce symptoms of the menopause, and it is also very nutritious. Eat one or two slices daily.

100g soya flour
100g wholewheat flour
100g porridge oats
100g linseed
50g sunflower seeds
50g pumpkin seeds
50g sesame seeds
50g flaked almonds
200g raisins
2pcs (approx 2 sq cm) grated fresh ginger
    or ½ teaspoon powder
½ teaspoon of ground nutmeg, cinnamon
1 tablespoon malt extract
750ml soya milk (this varies somewhat,
    have a 1 litre carton available)

(Makes 2 Cakes)

Mix all ingredients together well and leave to soak for 90 minutes.
If mixture is too stiff add more soya milk.
Line and grease two rectangular loaf tins.
Divide mixture between tins, bake for 60-90 minutes at 180°C.
Turn out and cool before eating. It freezes well.

# Detox Diet

This cleansing diet is a 10-day programme that is suitable if you are basically healthy but want to clear your system out and give your liver a chance to regenerate.

If you have a particular health problem you should have a consultation with a naturopath before going on a special diet.

This detox diet should be carried out at least once a year and preferably twice a year. Spring and autumn are traditional times to undertake a detox.

### DAY 1
Fruit for breakfast, lunch and in the evening. Choose one fruit for each meal from the following: apples, pears, kiwi fruit, grapes. Eat as much fruit as you like at one sitting.

### DAY 2, 3, 4, 5 AND 6
Fruit for breakfast. For lunch make a mixture of at least five salad vegetables: mix grated roots, sprouts and leafy vegetables.

In the evening eat cooked vegetables. Make a soup by boiling a mixture of at least five vegetables. Do not add any salt or seasoning. You may add fresh, chopped herbs or a handful of mixed seeds.

### DAY 7, 8 AND 9
Breakfast as day 2. Lunch as day 2 but in addition eat two rice cakes or two rye crispbreads. Evening as day 2 with the addition of a portion of brown rice or millet.

### DAY 10
Breakfast as day 2. Lunch as day 7. Evening as day 2 but in addition eat a baked potato with a small knob of butter (it will taste delicious!)

## Notes to Detox Diet

Drink lots of mineral water every day. Obtain as many as possible of the fruit and vegetables organically produced. Important things to avoid altogether throughout the diet are: tea, coffee, smoking, salt, pepper, recreational and non-essential prescription drugs and late nights.

A simple salad dressing, made by combining olive oil, lemon and fresh chopped herbs, may be added to the salad lunch.

## Snacks

- Mid-morning you can have an additional portion of fruit or a fruit smoothie.
- Mid-afternoon you can have a handful of roasted seeds e.g. pumpkin, sunflower or sesame seeds. Do not add salt.

# Symptoms Checklist

Some symptoms of the menopause can be confused with other, maybe more serious complaints. This checklist will help you to work out what your symptoms may be connected with, and remember if you are in any doubt at all then visit a qualified practitioner.

| SYMPTOM | OTHER POSSIBILITIES | MAIN DIFFERENCES |
|---|---|---|
| Hot flushes | Over-active thyroid | *Hyperthyroidism symptoms include flushing, sweating, palpitations, sleeplessness and weight loss. Symptoms will not respond to simple menopause treatments.* |
| Irregular periods | Fibroids, cancer | *Periods often become more erratic during the menopause before tailing off altogether but the following symptoms should be checked out:*<br>– *Very heavy periods or containing clots*<br>– *Bleeding after intercourse*<br>– *Periods lasting more than 7 days*<br>– *Fewer than 21 days between periods*<br>– *Any bleeding after the menopause is finished* |
| Palpitations | Over-active thyroid, heart disease, anaemia | *See hot flushes above for other symptoms of hyperthyroidism, anaemia is also likely to have symptoms of shortness of breath and tiredness in addition to palpitations.* |
| Depression and/or mood swings | Under-active thyroid, clinical depression | *Symptoms of hypothyroidism include weight gain, constipation, hair loss, dry/puffy skin, tiredness in addition to depression. If your mood swings are extreme or include social withdrawal, ongoing insomnia, disinterest in life or suicidal thoughts then seek professional advice.* |
| Bloated abdomen | Ovarian cancer | *Most women over 50 will find their waistline harder to keep trim but any unusual swelling or bloating in the abdomen should be checked out immediately.* |

# References

**Bibliography**
Curtis, S., "Essential Oils", 1996, Haldane Mason: London
Curtis, S., and Fraser, R., "Natural Healing for Women", 2003, Thorsons: London
Kenton. L., "Passage to Power", 1998, Vermilion
McIntyre, A., "The Complete Woman's Herbal", 1988, Gaia
Murray, M., Pizzorno, J., "Encyclopaedia of Natural Medicine", 1990, Little, Brown: London.
Northrup, C., "Women's Bodies Women's Wisdom", 1998, Piatkus: London.

**Where you can purchase products listed in this booklet**
You can obtain most of the products mentioned from Neal's Yard Remedies shops or mail order. See *www.nealsyardremedies.com* or *Tel: 0845 262 3145*

**Supplements**
Viridian Nutrition – *www.viridian-nutrition.com, Tel: +44 (0)1327 878050*

**Homœopathic Remedies**
Helios Homœopathic Pharmacy – *www.helios.co.uk, Tel: 01892 537254*
Ainsworth's Homœopathic Pharmacy – *Tel: 020 7935 5330, www.ainsworths.com*

**Finding a practitioner and organizations that can help**
Neal's Yard Remedies has Therapy Rooms with qualified practitioners throughout the UK. See *www.nealsyardremedies.com* or *Tel: 0845 262 3145*
It is important to find a practitioner that is fully qualified.
Listed below are organisations that can help you:
The Society of Homeopaths, *www.homeopathy-soh.org, Tel: 0845 450 6611*
Alliance of Registered Homeopaths, *www.a-r-h.org, Tel: 08700 736339*
British Association for Applied Nutrition and Nutritional Therapy, *www.bant.org.uk, Tel: 08706 061284*
The National Institute of Medical Herbalists, *www.nimh.org.uk, Tel: 01392 426022*
The General Council and Register of Naturopaths *www.naturopathy.org.uk, Tel: 01458 840072*
The Aromatherapy Consortium *www.aromatherapycouncil.co.uk, Tel: 0870 774 3477*

**Hormonal Testing**
This can be carried out by using kinesiology or by sending a sample to a laboratory for more detail. A number of practitioners in Neal's Yard Remedies Therapy Rooms offer this. *Contact Neal's Yard Remedies, Customer Services:*
*t: 01747 834634   cservices@nealsyardremedies.com*

## THE UNDERSTANDING SERIES

**Titles in the series:**
STRESS – Natural Solutions that Really Work, *by Susan Curtis*
ECZEMA – Natural Solutions that Really Work, *by Adrianna Holman*
DEPRESSION – Natural Solutions that Really Work, *by Dr Stephen Gascoigne*
MMR – The Facts, Choices and Alternatives, *by Lara Sussman*
THE MENOPAUSE – Natural Alternatives to HRT, *by Susan Curtis*
MEN'S VITALITY – Natural Solutions that Really Work, *by Tom Mettyear*

**Forthcoming:**
BACK PAIN – Natural Solutions that Really Work
INSOMNIA – Natural Solutions that Really Work
IBS – Natural Solutions that Really Work
AGEING – Natural Solutions that Really Work
ME – Natural Solutions that Really Work
CANDIDA – Natural Solutions that Really Work

SERIES EDITOR – Susan Curtis (RSHom)

**Author Biography**
Susan Curtis (RSHom) has been working with natural medicines for over 25 years. She originally trained as a homœopath, and has also studied and become an expert in the use of other forms of natural healing including essential oils and flower remedies.
Susan runs a busy natural health practice at Neal's Yard Therapy Rooms in Covent Garden, as well as writing and teaching about natural medicine.